# Beginners Guide to Obesity Using Diet

## Understanding the Importance of Diet in Obesity

By

Dunny Gilroy

# Table of Contents

# CHAPTER 1

# Introduction

Obesity, in recent decades, has emerged as one of the most pressing public health challenges globally. It is a complex, multifactorial condition characterized by an excessive accumulation of body fat, resulting in adverse health effects.

## 1.1 Understanding the Obesity Epidemic

**The Rising Prevalence of Obesity:** The obesity epidemic is not a mere exaggeration; it's a stark reality. Over the past few decades, the prevalence of obesity has surged to alarming levels, affecting people of all ages, races, and socioeconomic backgrounds.

**Health Implications of Obesity:** Obesity is not just about appearance; it's a major risk factor for a myriad of chronic health conditions.

**Causes and Contributing Factors:** Obesity is a complex interplay of genetic, environmental, and behavioral factors. dissect the root causes, such as genetics, environment, sedentary lifestyles, and societal influences, shedding light on why it's such a pervasive issue.

**Socioeconomic Disparities:** examine the socioeconomic disparities in obesity rates, discussing how income, education, and access to healthcare can influence one's risk of obesity. This insight highlights the need for a holistic approach to addressing the epidemic.

## 1.2 The Role of Diet in Obesity

**Diet as a Key Determinant:** The fundamental role of diet in the development and management of obesity. Diet is not just a contributing factor; it's often the primary driver of excess body weight.

**Caloric Balance:** At the core of the diet-obesity relationship is the concept of caloric balance. obesity results from an energy imbalance, where the number of calories consumed exceeds the number of calories expended. This balance is influenced by diet choices.

**The Western Diet and Processed Foods:** The modern Western diet, characterized by high levels of processed foods, added sugars, and unhealthy fats. This diet pattern has been closely linked to the obesity epidemic.

**Nutrition and Health:** It's not just about calories; it's also about nutrition. The importance of a well-balanced diet rich in essential nutrients and the role of micronutrients, such as vitamins and minerals, in maintaining overall health while managing weight.

**Eating Behaviors:** Beyond the content of our diets, we will explore eating behaviors and patterns. Topics include mindful eating, emotional eating, and the impact of social and cultural factors on dietary choices. Understanding these aspects can

empower individuals to make
healthier food decisions.

**The Promise of Dietary
Interventions:** dietary interventions
in tackling obesity. From low-carb
diets to plant-based diets and
intermittent fasting, there are various
dietary strategies that have shown
efficacy in weight management.

# CHAPTER 2

# The Basics of Obesity

## 2.1 What is Obesity

**Defining Obesity:** Obesity is not merely an issue of carrying excess weight; it's a complex medical condition. typically characterized by an elevated Body Mass Index (BMI), which reflects an individual's weight relative to their height.

**Stages of Obesity:** Obesity is not a one-size-fits-all condition. The various stages of obesity, from mild to severe, and the differences in health implications at each stage. Understanding these distinctions is vital for effective management.

## 2.2 Causes and Risk Factors

**Genetic Predisposition:** Genetics plays a significant role in obesity. The hereditary factors that can predispose individuals to obesity and how understanding one's genetic background can inform their approach to weight management.

**Environmental Influences:** Obesity is closely tied to the environment in which we live. The impact of the obesogenic environment, including factors like easy access to high-calorie foods, sedentary lifestyles, and the built environment that can promote or deter physical activity.

**Behavioral Factors:** Our behaviors, including eating habits, physical activity levels, and sleep patterns, contribute significantly to obesity.

behavioral risk factors and provide insights into making positive changes.

**Psychological Factors:** Emotional and psychological factors can also influence eating behaviors and weight gain. how stress, depression, and other mental health issues can contribute to obesity and strategies for addressing them.

# 2.3 Health Consequences of Obesity

**Systemic Health Impact:** Obesity is not just about excess weight; it affects nearly every organ system in the body. The systemic health consequences, including cardiovascular disease, diabetes, hypertension, and the increased risk of stroke.

**Metabolic Disturbances:** Obesity often leads to metabolic disturbances such as insulin resistance and dyslipidemia. These disturbances can exacerbate health issues and how they relate to diet.

**Psychosocial Effects:** Obesity can have profound psychosocial effects, including lower self-esteem, depression, and social stigma The importance of mental well-being in the context of obesity and its management.

# 2.4 Why Diet Matters

**The Role of Diet in Weight Gain:** To understand why diet matters in obesity, How the types and quantities of foods consumed directly influence body weight. The concept of caloric balance is revisited in this context.

**The Power of Dietary Change:**
Emphasizes that diet is not just a contributor to obesity; it's also a powerful tool for its management. The evidence supporting dietary interventions for weight loss and health improvement.

**Personalized Nutrition:** There is no one-size-fits-all diet for obesity. The concept of personalized nutrition, highlighting that individualized dietary approaches are often more effective and sustainable.

However, we also acknowledge the importance of incorporating other lifestyle changes, including physical activity and sleep.

# CHAPTER 3

# Getting Started with a Diet for Obesity

## 3.1 Assessing Your Current Diet

**Keeping a Food Diary:** One of the first steps in addressing obesity is gaining awareness of your current dietary habits.

**Identifying Problematic Patterns:** This includes recognizing high-calorie, low-nutrient foods and understanding emotional or mindless eating triggers.

**Nutrient Analysis:** This involves assessing your intake of macronutrients (carbohydrates, proteins, fats) and micronutrients (vitamins, minerals) to identify areas for improvement.

## 3.2 Setting Realistic Goals

**Understanding Goal Setting:** Effective goal setting is crucial for sustainable weight management.

**Non-Scale Goals:** Beyond the number on the scale, we encourage you to set non-scale goals related to health, fitness, and well-being. These can include improved energy levels, better sleep, or achieving physical fitness milestones.

## 3.3 Building a Support System

**The Role of Support:** Embarking on a diet for obesity can be challenging, and having a support system can make a significant difference.

**Professional Guidance:** In some cases, seeking guidance from healthcare professionals, such as dietitians or nutritionists, may be necessary.

**Online Communities and Resources:** With the advent of technology, there are numerous online communities, apps, and resources dedicated to supporting individuals in their weight management journey.

# 3.4 Common Dieting Pitfalls

While embarking on a diet for obesity can be a positive step towards better health, it's important to be aware of common pitfalls that individuals often encounter along the way. Understanding these challenges can help you navigate your weight loss journey more effectively and avoid potential setbacks.

**Extreme Dieting:** One of the most common pitfalls is embracing extreme or fad diets that promise rapid weight loss.

**Overly Restrictive Eating:** Restricting certain food groups or severely cutting calories can lead to feelings of deprivation and ultimately result in binge eating.

**Lack of Sustainability:** Many diets are challenging to sustain over the long term.

**Impatience:** Weight loss is a gradual process, and impatience can be a significant pitfall.

**Emotional Eating:** Emotional eating, using food to cope with stress, sadness, or boredom, is a common hurdle in weight management.

**Lack of Planning:** Failure to plan meals and snacks can lead to impulsive, unhealthy choices.

**Inadequate Hydration:** Dehydration can sometimes be mistaken for hunger, leading to unnecessary calorie consumption.

**Ignoring Portion Control:** Even healthy foods can contribute to weight gain if consumed in excessive quantities.

**Social Pressures:** Social situations and peer pressure can make it challenging to adhere to a healthy diet.

**Relying Solely on Diet:** While diet is a crucial component of weight management, neglecting physical activity can be a pitfall.

**Plateaus and Discouragement:** Weight loss plateaus are common and can be discouraging.

**Lack of Flexibility:** Being overly rigid in your dietary approach can lead to frustration and setbacks. We encourage flexibility in your diet and the ability to adapt to changing circumstances without derailing your progress.

Being aware of these common dieting pitfalls, you can proactively address and overcome challenges on your weight loss journey. Remember that making sustainable, gradual changes to your diet and lifestyle is more likely to lead to lasting success in managing obesity and achieving better health.

# CHAPTER 4

# Understanding Macronutrients

## 4.1 Carbohydrates

**What Are Carbohydrates:**
Carbohydrates are one of the primary macronutrients and serve as the body's primary source of energy.

**Types of Carbohydrates:**
Carbohydrates come in various forms, including simple carbohydrates (sugars) and complex carbohydrates (starches and fiber).

**Carbohydrates and Obesity:**
Carbohydrate consumption can play a significant role in obesity.

**Fiber and Satiety:** Dietary fiber is a crucial component of carbohydrates that contributes to feelings of fullness and aids in weight management.

**Recommended Carbohydrate Intake:** We provide guidelines for determining your daily carbohydrate needs based on factors like age, activity level, and overall health goals. This information helps you make informed decisions about carbohydrate consumption.

# 4.2 Proteins

**The Role of Proteins:** Proteins are essential for a variety of bodily functions, including building and repairing tissues, producing enzymes and hormones, and maintaining a strong immune system.

**Sources of Protein:** Protein can be obtained from both animal and plant sources.

**Proteins and Satiety:** Protein-rich foods are known to promote feelings of fullness and satiety, which can be advantageous in controlling calorie intake and managing weight.

**Protein Quality:** Protein quality matters, The concept of complete and incomplete proteins. Understanding protein quality helps you make choices that ensure you receive all essential amino acids in your diet.

**Protein Needs for Weight Management:** protein intake when aiming to manage obesity. Adequate protein consumption can help preserve muscle mass while promoting fat loss.

understanding the roles of carbohydrates and proteins in your diet, you can make informed choices that support your weight management goals. These macronutrients play a critical role in providing energy, promoting satiety, and ensuring your body gets the essential nutrients it needs to function optimally.

# 4.3 Fats

Fats, often misunderstood, are a vital macronutrient with significant implications for both health and weight management.

**Types of Dietary Fats:** Fats can be categorized into saturated fats, unsaturated fats (monounsaturated and polyunsaturated), and trans fats.

**Calories in Fats:** Fats are calorie-dense, containing more calories per gram than carbohydrates and proteins. The role of dietary fat in calorie consumption and why moderation is essential, especially when managing weight.

**Essential Fatty Acids:** Some fats are considered essential because your body cannot produce them on its own. The importance of essential fatty acids, such as omega-3 and omega-6, in maintaining overall health and managing inflammation.

**Fats and Satiety:** Like proteins, certain fats can promote feelings of fullness and satiety, potentially helping to control appetite and calorie intake.

**Choosing Healthy Fats:** Making informed choices about dietary fats is crucial.

# 4.4 How Macronutrients Affect Weight

**Caloric Balance Revisited:** We revisit the concept of caloric balance, emphasizing how the three macronutrients—carbohydrates, proteins, and fats—affect your overall calorie intake. Achieving the right balance of these macronutrients is essential for weight management.

**Impact of Carbohydrates:** Carbohydrates provide readily available energy, but their excessive consumption, particularly from sugars and refined sources, can lead to weight gain due to their effect on blood sugar levels and insulin responses.

**Role of Proteins:** Proteins play a vital role in preserving lean muscle mass during weight loss, which can be crucial for maintaining a higher metabolism. Adequate protein intake can support fat loss while preserving lean body mass.

**Fats and Satiety:** Dietary fats, especially healthy fats, contribute to satiety and can help control overall calorie intake. Including fats in your diet can lead to a greater sense of fullness, potentially reducing the urge to overeat.

**Balancing Macronutrients:** Achieving a well-balanced diet that aligns with your caloric needs and health objectives is key to effective weight management.

Understanding how macronutrients—carbohydrates, proteins, and fats—affect your body and weight is crucial for making informed dietary choices. Balancing these nutrients in your diet, along with considering calorie intake, is essential for achieving and maintaining a healthy weight.

# CHAPTER 5

# Creating a Balanced Diet Plan

Creating a balanced diet plan is a cornerstone of effective weight management and overall health.

## 5.1 The Importance of Balance

**Balancing Macronutrients:** Achieving a balance between carbohydrates, proteins, and fats is essential for providing your body with the necessary nutrients while managing calorie intake.

**Micronutrients and Nutrient Density:** Beyond macronutrients, The importance of micronutrients (vitamins and minerals) and the concept of nutrient density. A balanced diet should not only meet calorie needs but also provide a wide array of essential nutrients.

**Fruits and Vegetables:** Fruits and vegetables are nutritional powerhouses, rich in vitamins, minerals, and fiber.

**Whole Grains:** Whole grains are an excellent source of complex carbohydrates and fiber.

**Protein Sources:** Balancing protein sources, both animal and plant-based, ensures you receive a variety of amino acids and nutrients.

# 5.2 Portion Control

**Understanding Portion Sizes:** Portion control is a fundamental aspect of managing calorie intake. provide insights into understanding portion sizes, including the difference between portion sizes and serving sizes.

**Tools for Portion Control:** practical tools and strategies for managing portion sizes, such as using measuring cups, visual cues, and smaller plates to help you control calorie consumption.

**Mindful Eating:** Mindful eating is a valuable practice for portion control. The principles of mindful eating, including savoring each bite, eating without distractions, and listening to your body's hunger and fullness cues.

**Balancing Treats:** We acknowledge that indulging in occasional treats is a part of a balanced diet.

Creating a balanced diet plan that incorporates a variety of nutrient-dense foods while practicing portion control is key to successful weight management and overall well-being. By striking the right balance and being mindful of portion sizes, you can enjoy a satisfying and sustainable approach to healthy eating.

# 5.3 Meal Planning

Effective meal planning is a practical strategy for maintaining a balanced diet and managing obesity.

**The Benefits of Meal Planning**

- **Portion Control:** Meal planning allows you to control

portion sizes and avoid overeating by preparing appropriate servings in advance.

- **Nutrient Balance:** Planning meals in advance enables you to ensure a balanced intake of macronutrients and micronutrients, meeting your nutritional needs.

- **Time and Convenience:** Meal planning can save time and reduce stress by having meals ready when you need them, especially during busy days.

- **Healthier Choices:** With a plan in place, you're less likely to opt for unhealthy, convenience foods or takeout, as you have nutritious options readily available.

## How to Create a Meal Plan

- **Set Goals:** Determine your dietary goals, whether it's weight loss, improved health, or specific nutritional requirements.

- **Choose Recipes:** Select recipes that align with your goals and dietary preferences. Look for balanced meals that include lean proteins, whole grains, and plenty of vegetables.

- **Create a Shopping List:** After selecting recipes, compile a shopping list with all the ingredients you need. This helps avoid unnecessary purchases and keeps you on track.

- **Prep Ahead:** Spend some time preparing ingredients or full

meals in advance. Pre-cutting
vegetables, cooking grains, or
portioning out meals can save
time during the week.

- **Stay Flexible:** While planning
  is essential, it's also important
  to remain flexible. Life can be
  unpredictable, so be open to
  making adjustments as needed.

# 5.4 Grocery Shopping for Health

Smart grocery shopping is a crucial
step in maintaining a healthy diet for
obesity management.

**Planning Before You Shop**

- **Create a List:** Start by making
  a detailed shopping list based
  on your meal plan. This helps

you stay organized and avoid impulsive purchases.

- **Eat Before You Go:** Shopping on an empty stomach can lead to less healthy choices. Eat a balanced meal or snack before heading to the store.

**Making Healthy Choices**

- **Shop the Perimeter:** In most grocery stores, fresh produce, lean proteins, and dairy are typically located around the perimeter. Focus on these areas for healthier options.

- **Read Labels:** Pay attention to food labels, looking for items lower in saturated and trans fats, added sugars, and sodium. Check the ingredient list for hidden additives.

- **Choose Whole Foods:** Opt for whole, minimally processed foods whenever possible. This includes whole grains, fresh fruits and vegetables, and lean proteins.

- **Frozen and Canned Options:** Don't overlook frozen or canned fruits and vegetables, which can be just as nutritious as fresh and have a longer shelf life.

**Staying Mindful**

- **Avoid Impulse Buys:** Stick to your shopping list and resist the urge to purchase unhealthy snacks or items not aligned with your dietary goals.

- **Be Mindful of Sales:** Sales and promotions can be enticing, but they often involve less healthy options. Evaluate these deals carefully before purchasing.

- **Check for Discounts:** Look for discounts or coupons on healthier options like whole grains, lean proteins, and produce.

By mastering meal planning and practicing mindful grocery shopping, you can create a supportive environment for your dietary goals in managing obesity. These practical strategies help you maintain a balanced diet, control portion sizes, and make healthier food choices, all of which contribute to successful weight management and improved overall health.

# CHAPTER 6

# The Best Foods for Weight Management

## 6.1 Lean Proteins

Protein is an essential nutrient that plays a significant role in managing obesity. Lean sources of protein provide numerous benefits for weight management, including satiety, muscle preservation, and efficient calorie burning.

**Benefits of Lean Proteins**

- **Satiety:** Lean proteins are known for their ability to promote feelings of fullness and reduce appetite, which can help control calorie intake.

- **Muscle Preservation:** Protein
  is essential for maintaining and
  repairing muscle tissue. When
  you're trying to lose weight,
  preserving lean muscle mass is
  crucial for a healthy
  metabolism.

- **Thermic Effect:** Protein has a
  higher thermic effect than
  carbohydrates or fats, meaning
  it requires more energy to
  digest and metabolize. This can
  boost calorie expenditure.

## Sources of Lean Proteins

- **Poultry:** Skinless chicken and
  turkey are excellent sources of
  lean protein. Avoid fried or
  heavily processed options.

- **Fish:** Fatty fish like salmon,
  trout, and mackerel provide

healthy omega-3 fatty acids along with protein.

- **Lean Meats:** Lean cuts of beef or pork, such as sirloin or tenderloin, can be part of a balanced diet when trimmed of visible fat.

- **Plant-Based Proteins:** Incorporate plant-based protein sources like tofu, tempeh, legumes (beans, lentils, chickpeas), and quinoa into your diet.

## 6.2 Fiber-Rich Foods

Fiber is an often-overlooked component of a healthy diet that can greatly assist in weight management. Fiber-rich foods provide a range of benefits, including enhanced satiety, improved digestion, and stable blood sugar levels.

## Benefits of Fiber-Rich Foods

- **Satiety:** Fiber expands in the stomach, creating a feeling of fullness, which can help you eat less and control calorie intake.

- **Stable Blood Sugar:** Fiber slows down the absorption of sugars, preventing rapid spikes and crashes in blood sugar levels, which can lead to cravings.

- **Digestive Health:** A high-fiber diet supports healthy digestion and regular bowel movements, reducing the risk of overeating due to discomfort.

## Sources of Fiber-Rich Foods

- **Whole Grains:** Choose whole grains like oats, brown rice, quinoa, and whole wheat pasta for increased fiber content compared to refined grains.

- **Fruits:** Berries, apples, pears, and citrus fruits are excellent sources of dietary fiber. Be sure to eat them with their skin when possible.

- **Vegetables:** Dark leafy greens, broccoli, carrots, and sweet potatoes are among the many fiber-rich vegetable options.

- **Legumes:** Beans, lentils, chickpeas, and split peas are not only rich in fiber but also provide plant-based protein.

- **Nuts and Seeds:** Almonds, chia seeds, flaxseeds, and sunflower seeds are nutritious, high-fiber additions to your diet.

Incorporating lean proteins and fiber-rich foods into your daily meals can significantly contribute to effective weight management. These foods promote satiety, help control calorie intake, and support overall health.

# 6.3 Healthy Fats

Healthy fats play a vital role in your diet, and they are an important component of weight management.

**The Importance of Healthy Fats**

- **Satiety:** Like proteins and fiber, healthy fats contribute to feelings of fullness and satiety, helping to reduce overall calorie intake.

- **Nutrient Absorption:** Certain vitamins, such as vitamins A, D, E, and K, are fat-soluble, meaning they are better absorbed when consumed with dietary fats.

- **Cell Function:** Fats are essential for the structure and function of cell membranes, hormones, and various bodily processes.

**Sources of Healthy Fats**

- **Avocado:** Avocado is a nutrient-dense source of healthy fats, fiber, and various vitamins and minerals.

- **Nuts and Seeds:** Almonds, walnuts, chia seeds, flaxseeds, and hemp seeds are rich in healthy fats, protein, and fiber.

- **Olive Oil:** Extra virgin olive oil is a staple in Mediterranean diets and provides monounsaturated fats along with antioxidants.

- **Fatty Fish:** Salmon, mackerel, sardines, and trout are rich in omega-3 fatty acids, which are known for their heart-healthy benefits.

- **Coconut Oil:** While it's high in saturated fat, coconut oil contains medium-chain triglycerides (MCTs), which may have unique metabolic effects.

- **Nut Butters:** Natural peanut butter, almond butter, and other nut and seed butters can be nutritious sources of healthy fats and protein.

# 6.4 Fruits and Vegetables

Fruits and vegetables are the cornerstone of a healthy diet, particularly when managing obesity. They provide essential vitamins, minerals, fiber, and antioxidants while being low in calories.

**Benefits of Fruits and Vegetables**

- **Low Calorie Density:** Fruits and vegetables are typically low in calories while providing a high volume of food, making them ideal for weight management.

- **Fiber Content:** The fiber in fruits and vegetables promotes satiety, aids in digestion, and helps control calorie intake.

- **Nutrient Density:** Fruits and vegetables are rich in vitamins, minerals, and antioxidants, providing essential nutrients for overall health.

## Tips for Incorporating More Fruits and Vegetables

- **Variety:** Aim to consume a variety of colorful fruits and vegetables to ensure you get a wide range of nutrients.

- **Fresh, Frozen, or Canned:** While fresh produce is ideal, frozen and canned options are convenient and can be just as nutritious.

- **Snacking:** Use fruits and vegetables as healthy snacks to satisfy cravings while keeping calorie intake in check.

- **Meal Additions:** Incorporate fruits and vegetables into your meals by adding them to salads, stir-fries, smoothies, and as side dishes.

- **Meal Planning:** Include fruits and vegetables in your meal planning to ensure you have them readily available for cooking and snacking.

Balancing healthy fats and incorporating ample fruits and vegetables into your diet are fundamental strategies for effective weight management. These foods not only provide essential nutrients but also contribute to feelings of fullness and satiety, helping you control calorie intake.

# CHAPTER 7

# Special Diets for Obesity

Managing obesity often involves adopting specific dietary approaches that align with individual preferences and health goals.

## 7.1 Low-Carb Diets

**Overview of Low-Carb Diets**

- **Reduced Carbohydrate Intake:** Low-carb diets restrict the consumption of carbohydrates, particularly refined sugars and starchy foods like bread, pasta, and rice.

- **Emphasis on Protein and Healthy Fats:** These diets typically prioritize protein sources like lean meats, fish, and eggs, along with healthy fats such as avocados, nuts, and olive oil.

- **Ketogenic Diet:** The ketogenic diet is an extreme form of low-carb eating that aims to induce a state of ketosis, where the body burns fat for fuel instead of carbohydrates.

## Effectiveness and Considerations

- **Weight Loss:** Low-carb diets are often effective for weight loss due to reduced calorie intake and improved satiety from protein and fats.

- **Health Implications:** Some low-carb diets may raise

concerns about nutrient deficiencies and long-term effects on heart health. Consultation with a healthcare professional is advisable.

# 7.2 Mediterranean Diet

**Overview of the Mediterranean Diet**

- **Plant-Centric:** The Mediterranean diet emphasizes plant-based foods such as fruits, vegetables, whole grains, legumes, and nuts.

- **Healthy Fats:** It includes moderate consumption of olive oil, which is rich in monounsaturated fats, along with fatty fish like salmon and sardines.

- **Moderate Protein:** Lean sources of protein like poultry and legumes are staples, and red meat is consumed in moderation.

**Effectiveness and Considerations**

- **Heart Health:** The Mediterranean diet is associated with improved heart health, reduced risk of chronic diseases, and sustainable weight management.

- **Overall Wellness:** It promotes a balanced and sustainable way of eating that can be enjoyed for the long term.

# 7.3 Plant-Based Diets

**Overview of Plant-Based Diets**

- **Variety of Options:** Plant-based diets emphasize foods derived from plants, including fruits, vegetables, grains, legumes, nuts, seeds, and plant-based protein sources like tofu and tempeh.

- **Flexibility:** These diets can range from vegetarian (no meat) to vegan (no animal products) and can accommodate individual dietary preferences and restrictions.

## Effectiveness and Considerations

- **Weight Management:** Plant-based diets can be effective for weight management due to their emphasis on nutrient-dense, lower-calorie foods.

- **Nutrient Considerations:**
  Careful planning is required to
  ensure adequate intake of
  essential nutrients, such as
  vitamin B12, iron, and calcium,
  especially in vegan diets.

- **Environmental and Ethical
  Considerations:** Plant-based
  diets align with sustainability
  and animal welfare concerns.

# 7.4 Intermittent Fasting

**Overview of Intermittent Fasting**

- **Fasting Periods:** Intermittent
  fasting involves alternating
  between periods of eating and
  fasting. Common methods
  include the 16/8 method (16
  hours of fasting, 8 hours of
  eating) and the 5:2 diet (five

days of normal eating, two days
of low-calorie fasting).

- **Calorie Restriction:**
Intermittent fasting often leads
to reduced calorie intake, which
can promote weight loss.

## Effectiveness and Considerations

- **Weight Loss:** Intermittent
fasting can be effective for
weight loss due to calorie
restriction during fasting
periods.

- **Adherence:** It may not be
suitable for everyone, and
adherence can be challenging.
Individual response to fasting
varies.

- **Health Monitoring:**
Consultation with a healthcare
provider is advisable, especially

if you have underlying health conditions.

These special diets offer different approaches to managing obesity and promoting overall health. The choice of diet should align with individual preferences, health goals, and the guidance of a healthcare professional. Additionally, it's essential to focus on long-term sustainability and a balanced approach to diet and lifestyle modifications.

# CHAPTER 8

# Exercise and Physical Activity

## 8.1 Complementing Diet with Exercise

- **Calorie Expenditure:** Exercise helps increase your daily calorie expenditure, supporting a calorie deficit necessary for weight loss.

- **Metabolism:** Regular physical activity can boost your metabolism, helping you burn more calories at rest.

- **Muscle Preservation:** Exercise, particularly resistance training, helps preserve lean muscle mass during weight loss, which can prevent a drop in metabolic rate.

- **Health Benefits:** Exercise offers numerous health benefits beyond weight management, including improved cardiovascular health, increased strength and flexibility, reduced stress, and enhanced mental well-being.

# 8.2 Types of Exercises for Weight Loss

- **Cardiovascular Exercise:** Activities like walking, jogging, cycling, swimming, and dancing increase heart rate and calorie expenditure, making them effective for weight loss.

- **Strength Training:** Resistance exercises, using weights or bodyweight, build lean muscle, which can increase metabolism and promote fat loss.

- **High-Intensity Interval Training (HIIT):** HIIT involves short bursts of intense exercise followed by brief periods of rest or lower-intensity activity. It can be a time-efficient way to burn calories and improve fitness.

- **Flexibility and Mobility:** Stretching exercises, yoga, and Pilates enhance flexibility, balance, and overall body function.

# 8.3 Creating a Workout Routine

- **Set Clear Goals:** Determine your fitness goals, whether it's weight loss, improved fitness, increased strength, or enhanced well-being.

- **Start Slowly:** If you're new to exercise, begin with moderate-intensity activities and gradually increase intensity and duration over time.

- **Variety:** Incorporate a variety of exercises into your routine to prevent boredom and overuse injuries. Cross-training can also be effective for weight loss.

- **Frequency:** Aim for at least 150 minutes of moderate-intensity aerobic exercise or 75

minutes of vigorous-intensity
aerobic exercise per week,
along with strength training on
two or more days.

- **Consult a Professional:** If you
  have underlying health
  conditions or are unsure where
  to start, consider consulting
  with a fitness professional or
  healthcare provider.

- **Listen to Your Body:** Pay
  attention to your body's signals,
  such as pain or fatigue, and
  adjust your workout routine
  accordingly. Rest and recovery
  are essential parts of a balanced
  exercise plan.

- **Stay Consistent:** Consistency
  is key to reaping the benefits of
  exercise. Create a schedule that

aligns with your lifestyle and goals.

- **Enjoyment:** Choose activities you enjoy, as you're more likely to stick with them in the long term.

Remember that while exercise is a valuable tool for weight management, it should be viewed as part of a holistic approach that includes a balanced diet, adequate rest, and other lifestyle factors. Combining dietary changes with a well-designed exercise routine can lead to better outcomes in your journey to manage obesity and improve overall health.

# CHAPTER 9

# Overcoming Challenges and Plateaus

Managing obesity is a journey that may involve various challenges and plateaus along the way.

## 9.1 Dealing with Cravings

- **Identify Triggers:** Recognize the situations or emotions that trigger cravings. Is it stress, boredom, or specific foods?

- **Practice Mindfulness:** When cravings strike, take a moment to pause and consider whether you're truly hungry or if it's an emotional craving.

- **Healthy Substitutes:** Have healthier alternatives on hand for your favorite indulgences. For example, opt for dark chocolate instead of milk chocolate.

- **Portion Control:** If you choose to indulge, practice portion control to satisfy your craving without overeating.

# 9.2 Handling Emotional Eating

- **Emotional Awareness:** Learn to identify your emotions and the role they play in your eating habits.

- **Alternative Coping Strategies:** Develop alternative ways to manage emotions, such as journaling, meditation, deep breathing, or engaging in a hobby.

- **Seek Support:** Share your emotional struggles with a trusted friend, family member, or therapist who can provide guidance and support.

# 9.3 Breaking Through Plateaus

- **Reevaluate Your Routine:** Plateaus often indicate that your body has adapted to your current diet or exercise routine.

Consider making adjustments, such as increasing exercise intensity or changing your dietary approach.

- **Track Your Progress:** Keep detailed records of your food intake, exercise, and measurements to better understand what might be causing the plateau.

- **Patience:** Plateaus are normal in weight loss journeys. Be patient and stay committed to your goals.

- **Consult a Professional:** If a plateau persists for an extended period, consult a healthcare provider or nutritionist for guidance.

# 9.4 Staying Motivated

- **Set Short-Term Goals:** Break your long-term goal into smaller, achievable milestones. Celebrate your successes along the way.

- **Find a Support System:** Share your journey with friends or join a weight loss group. A supportive community can provide motivation and accountability.

- **Reward Yourself:** Treat yourself to non-food rewards when you reach your goals or achieve small victories.

- **Visualize Success:** Imagine yourself reaching your desired weight and visualize the positive changes it will bring to your life.

- **Adapt and Reevaluate:** If you find that your initial approach isn't working as expected, be open to adjusting your strategies and seeking new sources of motivation.

Overcoming challenges and plateaus is a natural part of the weight management process. With determination, self-awareness, and a willingness to adapt, you can successfully navigate these hurdles and continue making progress toward your health and weight goals.

# CHAPTER 10

# Tracking Progress

Tracking your progress is a valuable aspect of managing obesity through diet and lifestyle changes.

## 10.1 The Importance of Tracking

- **Accountability:** Tracking helps hold you accountable for your actions and adherence to your weight management plan.

- **Visibility:** It provides a clear picture of your progress, allowing you to identify areas that need adjustment.

- **Motivation:** Seeing your achievements and milestones

can boost motivation and reinforce your commitment to your goals.

- **Problem Solving:** If you encounter challenges or plateaus, tracking can help you identify potential reasons and make necessary changes.

# 10.2 Monitoring Weight and Measurements

- **Regular Weigh-Ins:** Weigh yourself consistently, such as once a week or every two weeks, at the same time of day and under the same conditions (e.g., after waking up and using the bathroom). This helps track trends over time.

- **Measurements:** In addition to weight, measure key areas like your waist, hips, and chest to track changes in body composition.

- **Progress Photos:** Take photos at regular intervals to visually document your transformation. These can be especially motivating when you compare them over time.

## 10.3 Keeping a Food Journal

- **Record Meals:** Document what you eat and drink, including portion sizes and details like preparation methods and ingredients. Be honest and thorough.

- **Note Emotions and Triggers:** In your journal, record how you were feeling when you ate and any emotional triggers for eating (e.g., stress, boredom).

- **Analyze Patterns:** Review your food journal regularly to identify trends, such as specific foods that trigger cravings or times of day when you tend to overeat.

- **Identify Successes:** Celebrate your victories by noting positive changes in your eating habits and choices.

# 10.4 Celebrating Milestones

- **Set Milestones:** Establish achievable short-term goals or milestones along your journey. These can be related to weight loss, fitness achievements, or other health markers.

- **Celebrate Achievements:** When you reach a milestone, celebrate your success. This could involve treating yourself to a non-food reward or simply acknowledging your progress.

- **Reflect on Progress:** Take time to reflect on how far you've come and the positive changes you've made to your lifestyle and health.

- **Stay Motivated:** Celebrating milestones reinforces your commitment to your goals and keeps you motivated to continue making progress.

Tracking progress, whether through weight and measurement monitoring, food journaling, or celebrating milestones, is a powerful tool in your obesity management journey. It provides insight, accountability, and motivation to help you stay on course and make adjustments when necessary.

# CHAPTER 11

# Maintaining a Healthy Weight

Maintaining a healthy weight is a long-term commitment that goes beyond initial weight loss.

## 11.1 Transitioning to Maintenance

- **Gradual Adjustments:** As you approach your goal weight, gradually transition from a weight loss-focused diet to one that supports maintenance.

- **Caloric Balance:** Find a balance between calorie intake and expenditure that allows you to maintain your weight without continuous weight loss.

- **Monitoring:** Continue monitoring your weight, measurements, and food intake, though with less frequency than during active weight loss.

# 11.2 Avoiding Weight Regain

- **Sustainable Habits:** Ensure that the dietary and exercise habits you've developed during your weight loss phase are sustainable in the long term.

- **Regular Exercise:** Maintain a consistent exercise routine to support metabolism and overall health.

- **Mindful Eating:** Continue practicing mindful eating, paying attention to hunger and fullness cues, and avoiding emotional eating.

- **Monitor Your Progress:** Regularly track your weight, measurements, and food intake to catch any signs of weight regain early and make necessary adjustments.

# 11.3 Long-Term Diet Strategies

- **Balanced Diet:** Maintain a balanced diet rich in whole foods, including lean proteins, whole grains, healthy fats, and plenty of fruits and vegetables.

- **Portion Control:** Continue practicing portion control to prevent overeating and maintain calorie balance.

- **Occasional Indulgences:** Allow for occasional treats and indulgences, but do so in moderation to avoid excessive calorie intake.

- **Stay Hydrated:** Adequate hydration is important for overall health and can support weight maintenance by reducing the likelihood of confusing thirst with hunger.

## 11.4 Embracing a Healthy Lifestyle

- **Regular Physical Activity:** Exercise should remain a

consistent part of your life. Find physical activities you enjoy to stay active.

- **Stress Management:** Continue to manage stress through techniques like meditation, yoga, or hobbies that bring you joy.

- **Sleep:** Prioritize sleep, as inadequate rest can disrupt appetite-regulating hormones and potentially lead to weight gain.

- **Social Support:** Maintain connections with a supportive community or friends who share your health and fitness goals.

- **Regular Health Check-ups:** Schedule regular check-ups with your healthcare provider to monitor your overall health and discuss any concerns.

Embracing a healthy lifestyle and maintaining a healthy weight is a lifelong commitment. It requires consistency, self-awareness, and a dedication to making choices that support your well-being. By following these strategies and maintaining a balanced approach to diet and exercise, you can increase your chances of long-term success in managing obesity and enjoying a healthier life.